A GUIDE TO COMMON KIDNEY PROBLEMS AND DISEASES

The Silent Impact of Infections on Vital Organs

SEAN T. ROLAND

COPYRIGHT

Copyright©2024 Sean T. Roland. All rights reserved. No part of this publication may be reproduced, distributed, or transmitted in any form or by any means, including photocopying, recording, or other electronic or mechanical methods, without the prior written permission of the publisher, except in the case of brief quotations embodied in critical reviews and certain other non-commercial uses permitted by copyright law.

TABLE OF CONTENTS

COPYRIGHT 2

TABLE OF CONTENTS 3

INTRODUCTION 5

  Common Kidney Problems and Diseases 5

CHAPTER 1 13

  Understanding Your Kidneys 13

CHAPTER 2 21

  Common Kidney Problems and Diseases 21

CHAPTER 3 31

  Warning Signs of Kidney Trouble 31

CHAPTER 4 41

  The Silent Threat: High Blood Pressure and Diabetes . 41

CHAPTER 5 53

  Diagnostic Tools and Tests 53

CHAPTER 6 65

  The Role of Diet in Kidney Health 65

CHAPTER 7 76

  Lifestyle Habits That Harm Your Kidneys 76

CHAPTER 8 88

Natural Remedies and Preventative Measures 88

CHAPTER 9 100

Living with Kidney Disease 100

CHAPTER 10 111

Healthier Lifestyle to Prevent Kidney Problems 111

CONCLUSION 123

Kidney Health Is a journey 123

INTRODUCTION
Common Kidney Problems and Diseases

The kidneys are among the most vital organs in the human body, silently working behind the scenes to keep us healthy and balanced. These two bean-shaped organs, located on either side of your spine just below the rib cage, perform functions that are nothing short of miraculous. Filtering toxins, balancing electrolytes, regulating blood pressure, producing hormones—your kidneys are at the heart of your body's well-being. Yet, for all the critical work they do, kidney health is often overlooked, with many people unaware of the risks until problems become serious.

Kidney diseases are alarmingly common, yet they often go unnoticed in their early stages. According to global health organizations, chronic kidney disease (CKD) affects one in ten adults worldwide, making it a significant public health concern. Even more alarming, millions remain undiagnosed, simply because the symptoms can be subtle or mistaken for other conditions. This lack of awareness and early intervention often leads to preventable complications, ranging from diminished quality of life to life-threatening kidney failure.

This book, *A Guide to Common Kidney Problems and Diseases,* aims to shine a light on these often-overlooked conditions. It is designed to educate, empower, and equip you with the knowledge you need to understand your kidneys, recognize warning signs, and take proactive steps toward prevention and management. Whether you are someone who has been recently diagnosed with a kidney condition, a caregiver for someone with kidney issues, or simply an individual interested in safeguarding your health, this guide will serve as your comprehensive resource.

Why Kidney Health Matters

Your kidneys do more than just process waste; they are central to maintaining overall health. They filter approximately 50 gallons of blood daily, removing waste products and excess fluids to produce urine. But their role extends far beyond filtration. They help regulate blood pressure by managing the balance of sodium and water in your body, produce the hormone erythropoietin to stimulate red blood cell production, and activate vitamin D to keep your bones healthy. When the kidneys fail to perform these functions effectively, the entire body feels the repercussions.

Kidney problems can manifest in various ways, ranging from mild discomfort to severe, life-altering conditions. Left untreated, even minor issues can escalate into chronic diseases, leading to complications such as heart disease, anemia, and weakened bones. Yet, many of these outcomes can be mitigated or avoided altogether with early detection and proper management.

The Silent Nature of Kidney Diseases

One of the most challenging aspects of kidney-related issues is their silent progression. Unlike other conditions that may present with obvious symptoms, kidney diseases often develop slowly, with few or no signs in the early stages. People may dismiss early symptoms, such as fatigue or swelling, as unrelated or insignificant. By the time symptoms become noticeable, significant damage may already have occurred.

This silent nature is why awareness is so critical. Regular checkups, including blood and urine tests, can detect early changes in kidney function. Simple tests like checking creatinine levels, glomerular filtration rate (GFR), and urine protein can provide invaluable insights into kidney health, allowing for timely interventions.

Common Kidney Problems and Diseases

The spectrum of kidney conditions is broad, ranging from acute issues like infections and kidney stones to chronic conditions like CKD and polycystic kidney disease (PKD). Some of the most common kidney problems include:

- **Chronic Kidney Disease (CKD):** A gradual loss of kidney function over time, often linked to diabetes, high blood pressure, or genetic predisposition.

- **Acute Kidney Injury (AKI):** A sudden decline in kidney function, often caused by dehydration, infections, or medication side effects.

- **Kidney Stones:** Hard mineral deposits that form in the kidneys and can cause excruciating pain.

- **Urinary Tract Infections (UTIs):** Infections that affect the bladder and kidneys, potentially leading to complications if untreated.

- **Polycystic Kidney Disease (PKD):** A genetic disorder causing fluid-filled cysts in the kidneys, leading to reduced function over time.

Each of these conditions presents unique challenges and requires tailored management strategies. Understanding the causes, symptoms, and treatments for these issues is the first step in taking control of your kidney health.

Risk Factors You Should Know

Several factors increase the likelihood of developing kidney problems. These include:

- **Chronic Conditions:** Diabetes and hypertension are the leading causes of kidney disease.

- **Family History:** Genetic predisposition plays a role in conditions like PKD.

- **Lifestyle Choices:** Smoking, poor diet, and lack of exercise can contribute to kidney problems.

- **Medications and Toxins:** Overuse of certain medications, such as NSAIDs, can harm the kidneys.

- **Age and Gender:** Kidney function tends to decline with age, and certain conditions are more prevalent in men or women.

Recognizing these risk factors allows for targeted prevention efforts. For instance, managing blood sugar levels in diabetics or encouraging hydration in individuals prone to kidney stones can make a significant difference.

Prevention is Key

While some kidney problems may be unavoidable due to genetics or other factors, many can be prevented through simple lifestyle changes. Staying hydrated, maintaining a balanced diet low in sodium and processed foods, exercising regularly, and avoiding tobacco are all steps that can reduce your risk of kidney disease. Regular health screenings are equally important, especially for those with risk factors like diabetes or hypertension.

Additionally, understanding the potential harm of over-the-counter medications, supplements, and environmental toxins is crucial. Many people unknowingly harm their kidneys by taking medications like ibuprofen or acetaminophen in excessive amounts or for extended periods. Educating yourself about these risks is one of the most powerful tools for protecting your kidney health.

Empowering You with Knowledge

The goal of this book is not only to inform but also to inspire action. Each chapter delves into a specific aspect of kidney health, from understanding the anatomy and function of these organs to exploring the latest advances in diagnosis and treatment. You will learn how to recognize early warning signs, navigate the healthcare system, and make informed decisions about your health.

This guide is also a call to action for adopting a proactive approach. Too often, people seek medical attention only when symptoms become severe. By prioritizing prevention and early detection, you can take control of your health and potentially avoid the complications of advanced kidney disease.

Looking Ahead

As you journey through this book, you will discover practical tips, expert insights, and real-life stories that illuminate the importance of kidney health. Whether it's understanding the impact of diet on kidney function or exploring the emotional challenges of living with a chronic condition, this guide aims to provide a holistic perspective on kidney wellness.

Remember, kidney health is a shared responsibility between you and your healthcare providers. By staying informed, you can work collaboratively to ensure that your kidneys continue to support you for years to come. Together, let's uncover the knowledge and strategies needed to protect these vital organs and improve overall well-being.

Your kidneys are the unsung heroes of your body. This book is your opportunity to give them the attention they deserve and take the first step toward a healthier future.

CHAPTER 1
Understanding Your Kidneys

Anatomy and Functions of the Kidneys

The kidneys are two bean-shaped organs located in the retroperitoneal space of your abdomen, one on each side of the spine. Each kidney is roughly the size of a fist and weighs about 4 to 5 ounces. Despite their small size, the kidneys perform a myriad of essential tasks that are critical for maintaining the body's internal balance and overall health.

Anatomy of the Kidneys

Each kidney is encased in a protective layer of fat and fibrous tissue called the renal capsule, which shields it from physical damage. Inside, the kidney is divided into three main regions:

1. **Cortex**: The outermost layer of the kidney where blood is filtered.

2. **Medulla**: The middle region, containing structures called renal pyramids that process filtered substances.

3. **Pelvis**: The innermost region where urine collects before being transported to the bladder via the ureters.

Blood enters the kidneys through the renal arteries, branches of the abdominal aorta, and leaves through the renal veins. Each kidney contains about one million nephrons, the microscopic structural and functional units responsible for filtering blood. Each nephron comprises:

- **Glomerulus**: A network of tiny capillaries that filter blood.

- **Bowman's Capsule**: A cup-like structure that collects the filtered fluid.

- **Tubules**: Tiny tubes that reabsorb essential nutrients and water while removing waste and excess substances.

Functions of the Kidneys

The kidneys are responsible for a wide range of functions essential to life. Their primary roles include:

1. **Filtration of Blood**: The kidneys filter approximately 50 gallons of blood daily, removing toxins, waste products, and excess fluids.

2. **Electrolyte Balance**: The kidneys regulate levels of sodium, potassium, calcium, and phosphate to maintain proper cell function.

3. **Acid-Base Balance**: They help keep the blood's pH within a narrow range by excreting hydrogen ions and reabsorbing bicarbonate.

4. **Blood Pressure Regulation**: By managing fluid levels and releasing the hormone renin, the kidneys play a pivotal role in controlling blood pressure.

5. **Erythropoiesis Stimulation**: The kidneys produce erythropoietin, a hormone that signals the bone marrow to create red blood cells.

6. **Vitamin D Activation**: They convert inactive vitamin D into its active form, which is essential for calcium absorption and bone health.

Why Kidney Health is Crucial for Overall Well-Being

The kidneys are integral to the proper functioning of almost every system in the body. When the kidneys are compromised, it can lead to a cascade of health problems that affect not just physical well-being but also mental and emotional health.

Maintaining a Stable Internal Environment

The kidneys' ability to filter and purify blood ensures that the body's internal environment remains stable. They remove urea, creatinine, and other waste products generated by cellular metabolism, preventing the toxic buildup that can lead to systemic issues.

Preventing Fluid Overload

Through the regulation of fluid balance, the kidneys prevent conditions such as edema (swelling caused by fluid retention) and hypertension (high blood pressure). This balance is crucial for the proper functioning of the cardiovascular system.

Supporting Cardiovascular Health

Healthy kidneys regulate blood pressure by controlling the volume of blood and the constriction of blood vessels. When kidney function declines, it often leads to uncontrolled hypertension, which increases the risk of heart attack, stroke, and other cardiovascular diseases.

Impact on Red Blood Cell Production

By producing erythropoietin, the kidneys ensure that the body maintains an adequate supply of red blood cells. A decline in kidney function can lead to anemia, characterized by fatigue, weakness, and a diminished ability to perform daily activities.

Preventing Chronic Conditions

Unhealthy kidneys can contribute to the development or worsening of chronic conditions such as diabetes and high blood pressure, creating a vicious cycle of deteriorating health. Conversely, maintaining kidney health can prevent these conditions or mitigate their effects.

The Role of Kidneys in Detoxification, Fluid Balance, and Hormone Production

The kidneys perform three primary roles that are essential for maintaining homeostasis: detoxification, fluid balance, and hormone production.

Detoxification

Every day, the kidneys process approximately 50 gallons of blood, removing waste products and toxins that accumulate from normal bodily functions, dietary intake, and environmental exposure. Key waste products include:

- **Urea**: Formed from the breakdown of proteins.
- **Creatinine**: A byproduct of muscle metabolism.

- **Excess Salts**: Sodium, potassium, and other electrolytes.
- **Toxins and Drugs**: Metabolized and excreted through urine.

The kidneys also neutralize and excrete acids generated during metabolism, which is vital for preventing acidosis, a condition that can disrupt cellular processes and lead to organ damage.

Fluid Balance

Maintaining the correct balance of fluids is one of the kidneys' most critical roles. By adjusting the amount of water excreted in urine, the kidneys ensure that the body remains neither overhydrated nor dehydrated. This balance affects:

- **Blood Pressure**: Fluid levels influence blood volume, which directly impacts blood pressure.
- **Cellular Function**: Proper hydration is essential for cells to carry out their functions efficiently.

In cases of dehydration, the kidneys concentrate urine by reabsorbing more water, whereas in cases of overhydration, they dilute urine to expel excess water.

Hormone Production

The kidneys produce and regulate several hormones that influence critical bodily functions:

1. **Erythropoietin (EPO)**: Stimulates the production of red blood cells in the bone marrow.

2. **Renin**: Plays a key role in the renin-angiotensin-aldosterone system (RAAS), which helps regulate blood pressure and electrolyte balance.

3. **Active Vitamin D (Calcitriol)**: Converts inactive vitamin D into its active form, aiding in calcium absorption and promoting bone health.

These hormonal functions underscore the kidneys' role as not just filters but also as endocrine organs that contribute to overall health and vitality.

Understanding the Impact of Kidney Dysfunction

When the kidneys are unable to perform their functions effectively, the repercussions can be far-reaching. Kidney dysfunction can lead to:

- **Toxin Accumulation**: Resulting in nausea, fatigue, confusion, and other symptoms.

- **Fluid Imbalances**: Causing swelling, high blood pressure, or dehydration.

- **Electrolyte Imbalances**: Leading to muscle weakness, irregular heart rhythms, and other complications.

- **Hormonal Deficiencies**: Causing anemia, weakened bones, and disrupted blood pressure regulation.

Understanding your kidneys is the first step toward appreciating their indispensable role in maintaining life and health. These remarkable organs are at the core of your body's ability to detoxify, balance fluids, and produce hormones essential for survival. By recognizing their significance and taking steps to protect them, you can ensure a healthier, more vibrant life.

CHAPTER 2
Common Kidney Problems and Diseases

The kidneys play a crucial role in maintaining overall health, but they are vulnerable to a variety of conditions that can significantly impact their function. From chronic kidney disease (CKD) to kidney stones and infections, understanding these issues is essential for prevention, early detection, and effective management. This chapter provides an extensive overview of common kidney problems, explores the risk factors and causes, and examines how lifestyle and genetics influence kidney health.

Overview of Conditions: Chronic Kidney Disease (CKD), Kidney Stones, and Infections

Chronic Kidney Disease (CKD)

Chronic kidney disease is a progressive condition characterized by the gradual loss of kidney function over time. CKD often goes undiagnosed in its early stages because symptoms are subtle or non-existent. By the time noticeable symptoms appear, significant damage may have already occurred. CKD is classified into five stages based on the glomerular filtration rate (GFR), a measure of kidney function:

- **Stage 1:** Kidney damage with normal or increased GFR (90 or above).
- **Stage 2:** Kidney damage with mild reduction in GFR (60-89).
- **Stage 3:** Moderate reduction in GFR (30-59).
- **Stage 4:** Severe reduction in GFR (15-29).
- **Stage 5:** Kidney failure (GFR less than 15), requiring dialysis or transplantation.

Common Symptoms of CKD:

- Fatigue and weakness.
- Swelling in the legs, ankles, or feet (edema).
- Persistent itching.
- Changes in urination patterns.
- Nausea or vomiting.
- Difficulty concentrating or confusion.

CKD is often linked to underlying health conditions, such as diabetes and hypertension. Early diagnosis and management are critical for slowing the progression of the disease.

Kidney Stones

Kidney stones are hard mineral and salt deposits that form in the kidneys. They can vary in size, ranging from tiny crystals to larger stones that cause significant pain and discomfort. Stones form when urine becomes concentrated, allowing minerals like calcium, oxalate, and uric acid to crystallize.

Types of Kidney Stones:

1. **Calcium Stones:** The most common type, formed from calcium oxalate or calcium phosphate.

2. **Uric Acid Stones:** Often associated with high protein diets or conditions like gout.

3. **Struvite Stones:** Linked to urinary tract infections (UTIs).

4. **Cystine Stones:** Rare and typically caused by genetic disorders.

Symptoms of Kidney Stones:

- Intense pain in the back, side, or lower abdomen.

- Hematuria (blood in urine).
- Nausea or vomiting.
- Frequent and painful urination.

Infections

Kidney infections, also known as pyelonephritis, are serious urinary tract infections that affect the kidneys. They often result from bacteria entering the urinary tract and ascending to the kidneys. If untreated, infections can lead to severe complications, including kidney damage or sepsis.

Common Symptoms of Kidney Infections:

- Fever and chills.
- Pain or burning during urination.
- Flank pain (pain in the side and back).
- Cloudy, foul-smelling urine.
- Fatigue and malaise.

Risk Factors and Causes of Kidney Problems

Several factors can increase the risk of developing kidney problems. Understanding these risk factors is crucial for implementing preventive measures and mitigating the likelihood of kidney disease.

Underlying Health Conditions

1. **Diabetes:**
    - High blood sugar levels damage the tiny blood vessels in the kidneys, impairing their ability to filter waste effectively.

2. **Hypertension:**
    - Chronic high blood pressure puts strain on the kidneys, leading to damage over time.

3. **Heart Disease:**
    - Cardiovascular conditions often coexist with kidney problems, as both share common risk factors.

4. **Obesity:**
    - Excess weight increases the risk of diabetes, hypertension, and metabolic syndrome, all of which can harm the kidneys.

Lifestyle Factors

1. **Dietary Habits:**
    - Diets high in sodium, sugar, and processed foods contribute to kidney damage.

- Insufficient hydration increases the risk of kidney stones and urinary tract infections.

2. **Smoking:**
   - Smoking reduces blood flow to the kidneys and accelerates the progression of CKD.

3. **Alcohol Consumption:**
   - Excessive alcohol intake can impair kidney function and exacerbate conditions like hypertension.

4. **Overuse of Medications:**
   - Nonsteroidal anti-inflammatory drugs (NSAIDs) and certain antibiotics can be toxic to the kidneys if used excessively or without medical guidance.

Genetic and Environmental Factors

1. **Family History:**
   - A genetic predisposition to conditions like polycystic kidney disease or Alport syndrome increases the risk of kidney problems.

2. **Ethnicity:**
   - Certain ethnic groups, such as African Americans, Hispanics, and Native Americans, have higher rates of kidney disease.

3. **Exposure to Toxins:**
   - Chronic exposure to heavy metals, chemicals, or pollutants can damage the kidneys.

Aging

Kidney function naturally declines with age. Older adults are at higher risk of developing CKD due to the cumulative impact of health conditions, medications, and lifestyle factors over time.

How Lifestyle and Genetics Impact Kidney Health

The Role of Lifestyle in Kidney Health

1. **Dietary Choices:**
   - A kidney-friendly diet emphasizes whole, unprocessed foods, lean proteins, and fresh fruits and vegetables while limiting sodium and potassium intake. Consuming enough

water is also crucial to maintaining proper hydration and preventing kidney stones.

2. **Exercise:**
   - Regular physical activity supports cardiovascular health and helps regulate blood pressure and blood sugar levels, both of which are essential for kidney health. However, overexertion can lead to dehydration, so staying hydrated is key.

3. **Hydration:**
   - Drinking adequate water helps the kidneys flush out waste and prevent the formation of kidney stones. Overhydration, on the other hand, can dilute essential electrolytes and stress the kidneys.

4. **Avoiding Harmful Substances:**
   - Limiting alcohol, avoiding recreational drugs, and moderating caffeine intake can reduce the strain on the kidneys.

5. **Sleep and Stress Management:**
    - Chronic stress and sleep deprivation negatively affect hormone levels, blood pressure, and overall kidney function.

The Role of Genetics in Kidney Health

While lifestyle choices play a significant role, genetics also influence kidney health. Individuals with a family history of kidney disease are more likely to develop related conditions. Genetic factors can:

- Predispose individuals to conditions like polycystic kidney disease or IgA nephropathy.
- Influence how the body processes and metabolizes certain substances, affecting kidney function.

Advances in genetic testing can help identify individuals at higher risk, enabling early interventions and personalized treatment plans.

Understanding common kidney problems and their underlying causes is the first step toward prevention and effective management. Chronic kidney disease, kidney stones, and infections are prevalent yet often preventable with the right knowledge and proactive measures. Risk factors such as diabetes, hypertension, and lifestyle habits significantly influence kidney health, while genetics also plays a role.

By making informed lifestyle choices and addressing underlying health conditions, individuals can reduce their risk of kidney problems and maintain optimal kidney function. Whether it's adopting a balanced diet, staying hydrated, managing stress, or seeking regular medical care, every effort contributes to healthier kidneys and a better quality of life. In the next chapter, we will delve deeper into recognizing the warning signs of kidney issues and exploring strategies for early intervention.

CHAPTER 3
Warning Signs of Kidney Trouble

The kidneys are essential to maintaining the body's internal balance, but they often suffer silently when problems arise. Kidney diseases are notorious for their subtle symptoms, which frequently go unnoticed until significant damage has occurred. Recognizing early warning signs is crucial for timely intervention and preventing severe complications. This chapter delves into the early indicators of kidney trouble, explores the subtle signs that might be easily overlooked, and underscores the importance of early detection for preserving kidney health.

Detailed Description of Early Symptoms

Changes in Urination

The kidneys are primarily responsible for filtering waste and excess fluids from the blood, excreting them through urine. Any change in urination patterns can be one of the earliest and most noticeable indicators of kidney problems. These changes might include:

1. **Increased Frequency:**
   - A need to urinate more often, especially at night (nocturia), could signal impaired kidney function or the presence of an infection.

2. **Decreased Output:**
   - Producing less urine than usual might indicate fluid retention due to declining kidney performance.

3. **Discoloration or Foaminess:**
   - Urine that appears darker, cloudy, or foamy may suggest the presence of blood, protein, or other abnormalities.

4. **Pain or Burning Sensation:**
   - Discomfort during urination could point to a urinary tract infection (UTI) or kidney stones.

Swelling (Edema)

The kidneys play a vital role in regulating fluid balance. When they fail to function properly, excess fluid can accumulate in the tissues, leading to swelling. This condition, known as edema, commonly occurs in the following areas:

- **Feet and Ankles:**
    - Swollen ankles or feet are among the most visible signs of fluid retention.
- **Face and Hands:**
    - Puffiness in the face, particularly around the eyes, is often a morning symptom of kidney dysfunction.
- **Abdomen:**
    - Severe kidney problems can lead to fluid buildup in the abdominal cavity, causing bloating.

Fatigue and Weakness

Healthy kidneys produce erythropoietin (EPO), a hormone that stimulates red blood cell production. When kidney function declines, the reduced EPO levels can result in anemia, leading to symptoms such as:

- **Persistent Fatigue:**
    - A lack of red blood cells to carry oxygen throughout the body causes extreme tiredness.
- **Shortness of Breath:**
    - Anemia can make even simple tasks feel exhausting.

Pain in the Lower Back or Sides

Pain localized in the lower back, sides, or below the rib cage may indicate:

- **Kidney Stones:**
    - Sharp, intense pain that radiates to the lower abdomen or groin.
- **Kidney Infections:**
    - Dull, persistent pain accompanied by fever and chills.

Other Physical Symptoms

1. **Nausea and Vomiting:**
    - A buildup of waste products in the blood can trigger gastrointestinal symptoms.

2. **Metallic Taste in the Mouth or Bad Breath:**
   - Toxins in the bloodstream may cause a metallic taste or ammonia-like breath odor.

3. **Dry, Itchy Skin:**
   - Imbalanced mineral levels or toxin buildup can lead to dryness and persistent itching.

Understanding Subtle Signs That May Go Unnoticed

Kidney diseases often progress silently, with symptoms that may be dismissed as minor inconveniences or attributed to other conditions. These subtle indicators are crucial to recognize:

Mild Changes in Energy Levels

Feeling slightly more tired than usual or noticing a decrease in stamina may seem insignificant but could signal early kidney dysfunction. This is particularly true if fatigue persists despite adequate sleep and rest.

Frequent Urinary Tract Infections (UTIs)

Recurring UTIs could indicate an underlying kidney problem, especially if accompanied by fever, back pain, or unusual urination patterns.

High Blood Pressure

Hypertension is both a cause and a consequence of kidney disease. Elevated blood pressure often develops silently and can exacerbate kidney damage if left untreated.

Loss of Appetite or Unexplained Weight Changes

A loss of appetite, accompanied by nausea or weight fluctuations, may result from toxins accumulating in the body due to declining kidney function.

Difficulty Concentrating or Confusion

Cognitive issues, such as trouble focusing or forgetfulness, may be related to anemia or the accumulation of toxins affecting brain function.

Foamy Urine

While foamy urine can occur occasionally due to dehydration, persistent frothiness might indicate protein leakage, a sign of kidney damage.

Why Early Detection Is Critical for Prevention

The earlier kidney problems are identified, the greater the chance of managing or reversing their progression. Early detection allows for timely interventions that can significantly improve outcomes and prevent complications.

Slowing the Progression of Kidney Disease

Early-stage kidney disease is often manageable with lifestyle changes, medications, and regular monitoring. Identifying issues before they advance can slow or even halt their progression, preserving kidney function.

Preventing Secondary Complications

When kidney problems are detected early, steps can be taken to avoid complications such as:

- **Cardiovascular Disease:**
    - Kidney dysfunction increases the risk of heart attack, stroke, and other cardiovascular events.

- **Fluid and Electrolyte Imbalances:**
    - Early management can prevent life-threatening imbalances.

- **Anemia and Bone Disorders:**
    - Treating underlying causes can alleviate symptoms and improve quality of life.

Reducing the Need for Advanced Treatments

Late-stage kidney disease often requires dialysis or a kidney transplant. Early detection can help patients avoid these invasive and life-altering treatments by preserving kidney function.

Empowering Patients to Take Control

Awareness and early detection empower individuals to make informed decisions about their health. Simple steps such as routine blood and urine tests can provide valuable insights into kidney function and help individuals take proactive measures.

The Role of Routine Screenings

Routine screenings are particularly important for individuals with risk factors such as diabetes, high blood pressure, or a family history of kidney disease. Key diagnostic tools include:

- **Blood Tests:**
    - Measure levels of creatinine and estimate the glomerular filtration rate (GFR).

- **Urine Tests:**
    - Detect proteinuria (protein in urine), hematuria (blood in urine), or other abnormalities.

- **Imaging Studies:**
    - Ultrasound or CT scans can identify structural abnormalities or blockages.

Promoting Preventive Health Measures

Detecting kidney issues early allows healthcare providers to recommend preventive measures tailored to an individual's needs, such as:

- **Dietary Modifications:**
    - Reducing sodium, protein, and phosphorus intake.

- **Hydration Strategies:**
    - Encouraging adequate water consumption to support kidney function.

- **Medication Adjustments:**
    - Prescribing drugs that protect the kidneys while avoiding potentially harmful ones.

The warning signs of kidney trouble often start subtly but can have far-reaching consequences if ignored. Changes in urination, swelling, fatigue, and other symptoms are key indicators that warrant immediate attention. By understanding the early and subtle signs of kidney dysfunction, individuals can take proactive steps to seek medical care, undergo diagnostic testing, and implement preventive measures.

Early detection is not just a medical necessity but a life-saving opportunity. Routine screenings, informed lifestyle choices, and timely interventions can make the difference between maintaining healthy kidney function and facing chronic disease or kidney failure. This chapter serves as a vital reminder to listen to your body and act on the warning signs to safeguard your kidney health and overall well-being. In the following chapters, we will explore practical strategies for preventing kidney problems and managing existing conditions effectively.

CHAPTER 4

The Silent Threat: High Blood Pressure and Diabetes

The kidneys are intricately connected to two of the most common chronic conditions affecting modern society: high blood pressure (hypertension) and diabetes. Both conditions pose a significant risk to kidney health, often working silently to cause damage over time. This chapter explores how hypertension and diabetes damage the kidneys, examines the connection between these chronic conditions and kidney failure, and provides actionable strategies for managing these conditions to protect kidney function.

How Hypertension and Diabetes Damage the Kidneys

Hypertension (High Blood Pressure)

Hypertension is one of the leading causes of kidney damage, primarily because it places excessive strain on the delicate blood vessels in the kidneys. These vessels, known as capillaries, are responsible for filtering waste products from the blood. Chronic high blood pressure causes these capillaries to weaken, thicken, or become damaged, leading to reduced kidney function.

Mechanisms of Damage:

1. **Increased Pressure on Blood Vessels:**
    - Elevated blood pressure forces the kidneys to work harder, increasing the risk of wear and tear on the filtering units (glomeruli).

2. **Reduced Blood Flow:**
    - Over time, narrowed blood vessels reduce the amount of blood reaching the kidneys, impairing their ability to filter waste effectively.

3. **Scarring (Nephrosclerosis):**
    - The kidneys' tiny blood vessels can become scarred, leading to permanent damage and reduced filtration capacity.

4. **Protein Leakage:**
    - Damaged blood vessels may allow protein to leak into the urine (proteinuria), an early sign of kidney dysfunction.

Diabetes

Diabetes is the most common cause of kidney failure, accounting for nearly half of all new cases in the United States. High blood sugar levels damage the kidneys in several ways, leading to a condition known as diabetic nephropathy.

Mechanisms of Damage:

1. **Hyperglycemia:**
    - Persistent high blood sugar levels damage the small blood vessels in the kidneys, impairing their ability to filter waste.

2. **Overworking the Filtering Units:**
    - High glucose levels force the kidneys to filter more blood than usual, putting extra strain on the nephrons (the kidney's filtering units).

3. **Oxidative Stress:**
    - Elevated blood sugar causes an increase in free radicals, which damage kidney cells and tissues.

4. **Inflammation:**
   - Chronic inflammation associated with diabetes exacerbates kidney damage by promoting scarring and fibrosis.

5. **Protein Leakage:**
   - Just as with hypertension, diabetes can lead to proteinuria, which indicates significant kidney damage.

The Connection Between Chronic Conditions and Kidney Failure

The Vicious Cycle of Kidney Damage

Hypertension and diabetes often coexist, creating a vicious cycle that accelerates kidney damage. For instance:

1. **Hypertension Worsens Diabetes:**
   - High blood pressure can increase insulin resistance, making diabetes more challenging to control.

2. **Diabetes Exacerbates Hypertension:**
   - High blood sugar levels cause the body to retain salt and water, leading to increased blood pressure.

3. **Combined Impact on the Kidneys:**
   - Together, these conditions significantly increase the risk of chronic kidney disease (CKD) and eventual kidney failure.

Progression to Kidney Failure

Kidney failure, or end-stage renal disease (ESRD), occurs when the kidneys lose nearly all their ability to function. Both hypertension and diabetes contribute to this progression in the following ways:

1. **Stage 1: Early Kidney Damage:**
   - Slight declines in kidney function with few or no symptoms. Proteinuria may be present.

2. **Stage 2: Moderate Damage:**
   - Symptoms such as fatigue, swelling, and changes in urination begin to appear.

3. **Stage 3: Severe Damage:**
   - Significant loss of kidney function with increased levels of toxins in the blood.

4. **Stage 4: Kidney Failure:**
   - The kidneys can no longer filter waste effectively, requiring dialysis or transplantation.

Impact on Other Organs

When the kidneys fail, the effects ripple throughout the body:

1. **Cardiovascular System:**
   - Kidney failure increases the risk of heart attack and stroke.

2. **Bones:**
   - Imbalances in calcium and phosphorus levels can weaken bones.

3. **Nervous System:**
   - Toxin buildup can cause neuropathy, cognitive decline, and seizures.

Managing Hypertension and Diabetes to Protect Kidney Function

Managing Hypertension

1. **Medications:**
   - **ACE Inhibitors and ARBs:**
     - These medications not only lower blood pressure but also protect kidney function by reducing proteinuria.
   - **Diuretics:**
     - Help remove excess fluid, reducing blood pressure and swelling.
   - **Calcium Channel Blockers:**
     - Relax blood vessels to improve blood flow.

2. **Dietary Changes:**
   - **Limit Sodium:**
     - Reducing salt intake lowers blood pressure and reduces fluid retention.

- Increase Potassium:
    - Foods rich in potassium, like bananas and spinach, can help balance sodium levels.
- Adopt the DASH Diet:
    - The Dietary Approaches to Stop Hypertension (DASH) plan emphasizes fruits, vegetables, whole grains, and lean proteins.

3. **Lifestyle Modifications:**
    - Regular Exercise:
        - Aerobic activity helps lower blood pressure and improve heart health.
    - Stress Management:
        - Techniques like yoga and meditation can reduce stress-related blood pressure spikes.
    - Quit Smoking:
        - Smoking damages blood vessels, exacerbating hypertension.

Managing Diabetes

1. **Medications:**

    o **Insulin and Oral Hypoglycemics:**

    - Essential for maintaining blood sugar levels within a healthy range.

    o **SGLT2 Inhibitors:**

    - A newer class of medications that protect kidney function by reducing glucose reabsorption in the kidneys.

2. **Dietary Changes:**

    o **Monitor Carbohydrate Intake:**

    - Focus on complex carbs with a low glycemic index to avoid blood sugar spikes.

    o **Limit Processed Foods:**

    - Reduce sugar and refined carbohydrates that can worsen diabetes.

- Stay Hydrated:
  - Proper hydration supports kidney function and reduces the risk of kidney stones.

3. Lifestyle Modifications:
   - Regular Monitoring:
     - Frequent blood sugar checks help maintain optimal levels.
   - Exercise:
     - Physical activity improves insulin sensitivity and blood sugar control.
   - Weight Management:
     - Maintaining a healthy weight reduces strain on the kidneys.

4. Routine Checkups:
   - Regular visits to a healthcare provider allow for early detection and management of kidney-related complications.

Collaborative Care

Effectively managing hypertension and diabetes requires a collaborative approach involving healthcare providers, dietitians, and patients. Key components of care include:

- **Individualized Treatment Plans:**
    - Tailored strategies address each patient's unique needs and risk factors.

- **Patient Education:**
    - Empowering patients with knowledge about their conditions and how to manage them.

- **Regular Monitoring:**
    - Routine blood pressure, blood sugar, and kidney function tests help track progress and adjust treatments as needed.

Hypertension and diabetes are silent but powerful threats to kidney health. Both conditions damage the kidneys in unique but overlapping ways, and their combined impact significantly increases the risk of chronic kidney disease and kidney failure. Understanding the mechanisms of damage and the connection between these chronic conditions and kidney health is essential for prevention and management.

Managing hypertension and diabetes is not just about controlling blood pressure and blood sugar levels—it's about protecting the kidneys and preserving overall health. Through a combination of medications, dietary changes, lifestyle modifications, and regular medical care, individuals can reduce their risk of kidney damage and improve their quality of life. By taking proactive steps and seeking collaborative care, patients can break the cycle of kidney damage and chronic disease, ensuring a healthier future.

CHAPTER 5
Diagnostic Tools and Tests

Diagnosing kidney problems accurately and early is crucial for effective management and treatment. The kidneys are silent workers, and their dysfunction often remains undetected until significant damage occurs. Diagnostic tools and tests play a pivotal role in identifying kidney health issues, assessing the severity of any problems, and guiding treatment plans. This chapter explores the types of tests available, interprets test results, and provides guidance on when to seek the expertise of a nephrologist.

Types of Tests: Blood Tests, Urine Tests, Imaging Studies, and Biopsies

Blood Tests

Blood tests are among the most common and reliable methods for assessing kidney function. They provide crucial insights into how well the kidneys are filtering waste products and maintaining the body's chemical balance.

1. **Serum Creatinine Test**
    - Creatinine is a waste product produced by muscle metabolism and excreted by the

kidneys. Elevated levels in the blood indicate reduced kidney function.

- **Normal Range:**
    - Men: 0.7 to 1.3 mg/dL
    - Women: 0.6 to 1.1 mg/dL
- **What It Indicates:** Higher levels suggest impaired filtration and possible kidney disease.

2. **Glomerular Filtration Rate (GFR)**
    - GFR measures how efficiently the kidneys filter blood. It is calculated using serum creatinine, age, sex, and race.
    - **Stages of Kidney Function:**
        - Normal: 90 mL/min or above
        - Mild reduction: 60-89 mL/min
        - Moderate reduction: 30-59 mL/min
        - Severe reduction: 15-29 mL/min
        - Kidney failure: Below 15 mL/min

3. **Blood Urea Nitrogen (BUN)**
    - Urea is another waste product filtered by the kidneys. Elevated BUN levels can indicate kidney dysfunction or dehydration.
    - **Normal Range:** 7 to 20 mg/dL

4. **Electrolyte Panel**
    - The kidneys regulate electrolyte levels, including sodium, potassium, calcium, and bicarbonate. Imbalances may signal kidney issues.

5. **Albumin Levels**
    - Albumin is a protein essential for maintaining fluid balance. Low levels in the blood could indicate protein leakage due to kidney damage.

Urine Tests

Urine tests provide a direct evaluation of kidney function and can detect abnormalities that indicate kidney disease.

1. **Urinalysis**
   - A basic test to check the appearance, concentration, and content of urine.
   - **Key Indicators:**
     - Cloudy urine may suggest infection.
     - Foamy urine could indicate protein leakage.
     - Blood in the urine (hematuria) may point to infections, stones, or glomerular diseases.

2. **Proteinuria Test**
   - Measures the amount of protein in the urine.
   - Persistent proteinuria is a hallmark sign of kidney damage.

3. **Microalbuminuria Test**
   - Detects small amounts of albumin in the urine, often an early indicator of kidney disease in people with diabetes or hypertension.

4. **24-Hour Urine Collection**
   - Provides a comprehensive analysis of kidney function by measuring waste products and protein levels over a 24-hour period.

5. **Creatinine Clearance Test**
   - Compares creatinine levels in blood and urine to evaluate how well the kidneys are filtering waste.

Imaging Studies

Imaging techniques help visualize the structure and size of the kidneys, detect abnormalities, and identify potential causes of kidney dysfunction.

1. **Ultrasound**
   - A non-invasive test that uses sound waves to create images of the kidneys.
   - **Uses:**
     - Detecting kidney stones or cysts.
     - Identifying blockages or structural abnormalities.

2. **CT Scan (Computed Tomography)**
   - Produces detailed cross-sectional images of the kidneys and surrounding structures.
   - **Uses:**
     - Identifying tumors, abscesses, or other abnormalities.

3. **MRI (Magnetic Resonance Imaging)**
   - Provides high-resolution images using magnetic fields and radio waves.
   - **Uses:**
     - Evaluating soft tissue and vascular abnormalities.

4. **Nuclear Medicine Scans**
   - Involves injecting a radioactive tracer to assess kidney function and blood flow.
   - **Uses:**
     - Measuring filtration rates.
     - Identifying kidney scars or blockages.

Biopsies

A kidney biopsy involves removing a small sample of kidney tissue for analysis. It is typically recommended when other tests are inconclusive or when specific diseases are suspected.

1. **Procedure:**
    - Performed under local anesthesia, a needle is inserted through the skin to collect a tissue sample.

2. **Uses:**
    - Diagnosing glomerular diseases, such as glomerulonephritis.
    - Assessing the extent of kidney damage.
    - Guiding treatment plans for kidney disease.

3. **Risks:**
    - Bleeding, infection, or discomfort at the biopsy site.

What Test Results Mean for Your Kidney Health

Normal vs. Abnormal Results

Interpreting test results requires understanding the normal ranges for various markers of kidney function:

- **GFR:**
    - A GFR above 60 mL/min is generally considered normal.
    - Below 60 mL/min for three months or more indicates chronic kidney disease.

- **Serum Creatinine:**
    - High levels suggest impaired filtration, but values may vary based on muscle mass, age, and gender.

- **Proteinuria:**
    - Persistent protein in the urine indicates damage to the glomeruli, the filtering units of the kidneys.

- **Blood Pressure:**
    - Elevated blood pressure is both a cause and a result of kidney dysfunction.

Patterns and Trends

Kidney health is best assessed by looking at patterns over time rather than single test results. For example:

- A steady increase in serum creatinine levels over months or years suggests progressive kidney dysfunction.
- Consistently high levels of protein in the urine may indicate worsening kidney damage.

Markers of Advanced Disease

- Severe reductions in GFR (below 15 mL/min) signify end-stage renal disease (ESRD), requiring dialysis or transplantation.
- Electrolyte imbalances, such as high potassium levels, may indicate life-threatening complications of kidney failure.

When to See a Nephrologist

A nephrologist is a specialist in kidney care. While general practitioners can address early-stage kidney concerns, certain situations warrant a referral to a nephrologist.

Signs That You Should Consult a Nephrologist

1. **Abnormal Test Results:**
   - Persistent proteinuria or hematuria.
   - Declining GFR or rising serum creatinine levels.

2. **Chronic Conditions:**
   - Uncontrolled diabetes or hypertension.
   - Conditions like lupus that may affect the kidneys.

3. **Severe Symptoms:**
   - Swelling (edema) that does not improve with treatment.
   - Persistent fatigue or unexplained weakness.

4. **Family History:**
   - A family history of kidney disease, such as polycystic kidney disease (PKD).

5. **Complications:**
   - Difficult-to-control blood pressure.
   - Signs of advanced kidney disease, such as confusion, nausea, or shortness of breath.

What to Expect During a Nephrologist Visit

1. **Comprehensive Evaluation:**
   - Review of medical history, current symptoms, and previous test results.

2. **Additional Tests:**
   - A nephrologist may order advanced diagnostic tests, such as a renal biopsy or imaging studies, to determine the cause and extent of kidney damage.

3. **Treatment Planning:**
   - Developing a personalized treatment plan, which may include medications, dietary changes, and lifestyle modifications.

4. **Monitoring and Follow-Up:**
   - Regular check-ups to monitor disease progression and adjust treatments as needed.

The Importance of Early Referral

Seeing a nephrologist early in the course of kidney disease can:

- Slow disease progression.

- Prevent complications.
- Reduce the need for dialysis or transplantation.

Diagnostic tools and tests are the cornerstone of kidney health management. Blood tests, urine analyses, imaging studies, and biopsies provide critical insights into the kidneys' structure and function, enabling early detection and timely interventions. Understanding what these tests reveal about your kidney health empowers you to take proactive steps to maintain or improve function.

Knowing when to consult a nep

hrologist is equally important. Early referral and specialized care can make a significant difference in the trajectory of kidney disease, preventing severe complications and preserving quality of life. By staying informed and vigilant, you can work with your healthcare team to protect these vital organs and ensure long-term health.

CHAPTER 6

The Role of Diet in Kidney Health

The health of your kidneys is deeply influenced by the food and beverages you consume. These vital organs filter waste, balance electrolytes, and regulate blood pressure, among many other essential functions. A kidney-friendly diet can preserve kidney function, prevent complications, and improve overall health. This chapter explores the foods that support kidney function, harmful foods to avoid, and the critical role hydration plays in maintaining kidney health.

Foods That Support Kidney Function

Certain foods can help maintain healthy kidneys by providing essential nutrients, reducing inflammation, and preventing the buildup of harmful substances. Incorporating these foods into your diet can support kidney function and protect against chronic kidney disease (CKD).

Low-Sodium Foods

Excess sodium can strain the kidneys, leading to high blood pressure and fluid retention. Opt for foods that are naturally low in sodium:

- **Fresh Fruits and Vegetables:** Apples, berries, carrots, cucumbers, and leafy greens.

- **Whole Grains:** Quinoa, brown rice, and whole oats.

- **Lean Proteins:** Skinless chicken, turkey, and eggs (in moderation).

- **Herbs and Spices:** Use garlic, basil, and rosemary as flavorful alternatives to salt.

Foods Rich in Antioxidants

Antioxidants protect the kidneys by neutralizing free radicals, which can damage cells and tissues. Include:

- **Berries:** Blueberries, strawberries, and raspberries.

- **Cruciferous Vegetables:** Broccoli, cauliflower, and Brussels sprouts.

- **Citrus Fruits:** Oranges, lemons, and grapefruits (in moderation, depending on potassium levels).

- **Dark Chocolate:** Rich in flavonoids, which may reduce inflammation and improve kidney health.

Low-Potassium Foods

For individuals with compromised kidney function, controlling potassium intake is crucial. Opt for:

- **Low-Potassium Fruits:** Apples, grapes, and cranberries.

- **Low-Potassium Vegetables:** Green beans, zucchini, and lettuce.

- **Refined Grains:** White rice and pasta (if whole grains are restricted due to potassium levels).

Omega-3 Fatty Acids

Omega-3 fatty acids reduce inflammation and may lower blood pressure, both of which benefit kidney health. Include:

- **Fatty Fish:** Salmon, mackerel, and sardines.

- **Flaxseeds and Chia Seeds:** Great plant-based sources of omega-3s.

Probiotic Foods

Probiotics help maintain a healthy gut microbiome, which can indirectly support kidney function by reducing toxin production. Examples include:

- **Yogurt:** Opt for low-sugar, low-potassium varieties.

- **Kefir:** A fermented milk drink rich in beneficial bacteria.

- **Fermented Vegetables:** Sauerkraut and kimchi (watch sodium content).

Harmful Foods to Avoid

Certain foods can harm kidney health by increasing the workload on these organs, contributing to imbalances, or promoting disease progression. Understanding which foods to limit or avoid is critical for maintaining kidney function.

High-Sodium Foods

Excessive sodium can lead to fluid retention and high blood pressure, both of which strain the kidneys. Avoid:

- **Processed Foods:** Canned soups, frozen meals, and packaged snacks.
- **Salty Snacks:** Chips, pretzels, and salted nuts.
- **Cured Meats:** Bacon, sausage, and deli meats.
- **Fast Food:** Burgers, fries, and pizza.

High-Potassium Foods

For individuals with CKD or impaired kidney function, excess potassium can be dangerous, leading to irregular heart rhythms or muscle weakness. Limit:

- **Bananas:** High in potassium and often restricted.

- **Avocados:** Although nutrient-dense, their potassium content can be problematic.
- **Tomatoes and Tomato Products:** Including sauces and soups.
- **Potatoes:** Opt for leaching techniques (soaking and boiling) if consumed.

High-Phosphorus Foods

Too much phosphorus can weaken bones and cause vascular calcification in those with kidney disease. Avoid:

- **Dairy Products:** Milk, cheese, and yogurt.
- **Processed Foods:** Contain phosphorus additives for flavor and preservation.
- **Cola Beverages:** High in phosphorus from additives.

Sugary Foods and Drinks

Excessive sugar intake contributes to obesity and diabetes, both of which increase the risk of kidney disease. Avoid:

- **Sugary Beverages:** Soda, energy drinks, and sweetened teas.
- **Desserts:** Cakes, cookies, and candies.

- **Sweetened Cereals:** Often loaded with added sugars.

Alcohol

Excessive alcohol consumption can impair kidney function by dehydrating the body and increasing blood pressure. Limit alcohol to moderate levels or avoid it entirely if you have kidney concerns.

Hydration and Its Role in Maintaining Healthy Kidneys

Hydration is fundamental to kidney health. The kidneys rely on adequate fluid intake to filter waste products, maintain electrolyte balance, and regulate blood pressure. Insufficient hydration can lead to kidney stones, infections, and other complications.

Benefits of Staying Hydrated

1. **Efficient Waste Removal:**
    - Water helps dissolve waste products and toxins, allowing the kidneys to expel them effectively through urine.

2. **Prevention of Kidney Stones:**
    - Proper hydration dilutes urine, reducing the concentration of minerals that form kidney stones.

3. **Urinary Tract Health:**
    - Drinking enough fluids flushes out bacteria, preventing urinary tract infections (UTIs).

4. **Blood Pressure Regulation:**
    - Adequate hydration supports healthy blood volume, which in turn helps regulate blood pressure.

How Much Water Is Enough?

The amount of water needed varies based on individual factors such as age, weight, activity level, and climate. General recommendations include:

- **Healthy Adults:**
    - About 8-10 cups (64-80 ounces) per day.
- **Individuals with Kidney Issues:**

- o Fluid intake may need to be adjusted based on specific conditions and a doctor's recommendations.

Signs of Proper Hydration

1. **Clear or Light Yellow Urine:**
   - o Indicates adequate hydration levels.

2. **Regular Urination:**
   - o Most people urinate 6-8 times per day when adequately hydrated.

3. **No Thirst:**
   - o Thirst is often a late indicator of dehydration.

Dehydration Risks

Dehydration forces the kidneys to work harder, increasing the risk of complications such as:

1. **Kidney Stones:**
   - o Concentrated urine promotes stone formation.

2. **Acute Kidney Injury (AKI):**

   o Severe dehydration can lead to a sudden decline in kidney function.

3. **Infections:**

   o Insufficient fluid intake increases the risk of UTIs, which can ascend to the kidneys (pyelonephritis).

Beverages to Avoid

Not all fluids are equally beneficial for kidney health. Limit:

- **Sugary Drinks:** Increase calorie intake without providing hydration benefits.

- **Caffeinated Beverages:** Excessive caffeine can act as a diuretic, leading to dehydration.

- **Alcohol:** Dehydrates the body and strains kidney function.

Combining Diet and Hydration for Optimal Kidney Health

A kidney-friendly diet and proper hydration work hand in hand to maintain kidney health. By focusing on nutrient-dense, low-sodium, and low-potassium foods and ensuring adequate water intake, you can:

- Support kidney function.
- Prevent complications such as kidney stones and infections.
- Reduce the risk of chronic kidney disease progression.

Practical Tips for a Kidney-Friendly Lifestyle

1. **Plan Balanced Meals:**
   - Incorporate a variety of fruits, vegetables, lean proteins, and whole grains while monitoring potassium, phosphorus, and sodium levels.

2. **Stay Hydrated:**
   - Carry a water bottle and drink regularly throughout the day.

3. **Read Labels:**
   - Look for hidden sodium, potassium, and phosphorus in processed foods.

4. **Consult a Dietitian:**
    - A registered dietitian can tailor dietary recommendations to your specific needs and medical conditions.

Diet and hydration are central to maintaining healthy kidneys. Foods rich in antioxidants, low in sodium, and balanced in potassium can support kidney function, while avoiding harmful foods and beverages can prevent further strain on these vital organs. Adequate hydration ensures efficient waste removal, prevents kidney stones, and supports overall urinary tract health.

By making informed dietary choices and prioritizing hydration, you can protect your kidneys and promote long-term well-being. Whether you are managing a chronic condition or aiming to maintain optimal health, your diet and hydration habits are powerful tools in supporting kidney health.

CHAPTER 7
Lifestyle Habits That Harm Your Kidneys

The kidneys are vital organs responsible for filtering toxins, maintaining fluid balance, and regulating blood pressure. However, certain lifestyle habits can severely compromise kidney function over time. Understanding these risks and adopting healthier habits can significantly improve kidney health and overall well-being. This chapter explores the effects of smoking, alcohol, and dehydration, the dangers of over-the-counter medications and supplements, and how stress and lack of sleep impact kidney health.

Effects of Smoking, Alcohol, and Dehydration

Smoking

Smoking is one of the most harmful habits for kidney health. It damages blood vessels, reduces oxygen flow, and increases the risk of chronic kidney disease (CKD).

1. **Impact on Blood Vessels:**
    - Smoking narrows and hardens blood vessels, impairing circulation to the kidneys. Reduced blood flow can compromise the kidneys' ability to filter waste effectively.

2. **Accelerated Kidney Damage:**
   - Smokers with pre-existing conditions like diabetes or hypertension are more likely to experience accelerated kidney damage compared to non-smokers.

3. **Increased Risk of CKD and Kidney Cancer:**
   - Studies show that smoking doubles the risk of developing CKD. Additionally, smokers are at higher risk for renal cell carcinoma, the most common type of kidney cancer.

4. **Reduced Effectiveness of Medications:**
   - Smoking can interfere with medications designed to manage kidney-related conditions, making treatment less effective.

Alcohol

Excessive alcohol consumption places a significant strain on the kidneys and can lead to acute or chronic kidney problems.

1. **Dehydration:**
   - Alcohol acts as a diuretic, increasing urine production and leading to dehydration.

Dehydration reduces kidney function and increases the risk of kidney stones.

2. **High Blood Pressure:**
   o Chronic alcohol use raises blood pressure, a leading cause of CKD.

3. **Toxin Overload:**
   o The kidneys must work harder to filter the toxins in alcohol, increasing their workload and potentially causing long-term damage.

4. **Risk of Acute Kidney Injury (AKI):**
   o Binge drinking can lead to sudden kidney failure, especially in individuals with pre-existing kidney conditions.

Dehydration

Dehydration is a common but often overlooked factor that can harm the kidneys. The kidneys rely on adequate water intake to filter waste and maintain electrolyte balance.

1. **Concentrated Urine:**
   o Insufficient water intake leads to concentrated urine, increasing the risk of

kidney stones and urinary tract infections (UTIs).

2. **Reduced Waste Elimination:**
   - Dehydration impairs the kidneys' ability to remove toxins, which can accumulate in the body and cause further harm.

3. **Chronic Dehydration:**
   - Over time, chronic dehydration can lead to kidney damage and contribute to CKD progression.

The Dangers of Over-the-Counter Medications and Supplements

Many people underestimate the impact of over-the-counter (OTC) medications and dietary supplements on kidney health. While these products are widely accessible, their misuse or overuse can have serious consequences.

Nonsteroidal Anti-Inflammatory Drugs (NSAIDs)

NSAIDs like ibuprofen, naproxen, and aspirin are commonly used for pain relief but can harm the kidneys when taken excessively or for prolonged periods.

1. **Reduced Blood Flow to the Kidneys:**

- NSAIDs inhibit the production of prostaglandins, hormones that help maintain blood flow to the kidneys. Reduced blood flow can lead to acute kidney injury (AKI).

2. **Risk of Chronic Kidney Damage:**
    - Long-term use of NSAIDs, particularly in high doses, increases the risk of CKD.

3. **Heightened Risk for Vulnerable Populations:**
    - Individuals with diabetes, hypertension, or pre-existing kidney disease are at greater risk of NSAID-related kidney damage.

Antacids and Proton Pump Inhibitors (PPIs)

Medications used to treat acid reflux and heartburn can also impact kidney health.

1. **Risk of CKD:**
    - Studies have linked long-term PPI use to an increased risk of CKD and kidney failure.

2. **Potential for Interstitial Nephritis:**
    - PPIs can cause inflammation of the kidneys, a condition known as interstitial nephritis,

which may lead to permanent damage if untreated.

Herbal Supplements

While often marketed as natural and safe, herbal supplements can pose risks to kidney health, particularly when taken without medical supervision.

1. **Unregulated Ingredients:**
    - Many supplements contain hidden ingredients or contaminants that can harm the kidneys.

2. **Toxic Herbs:**
    - Certain herbs, such as aristolochia and cascara, are known to cause kidney damage.

3. **Excessive Nutrient Load:**
    - Supplements high in potassium, phosphorus, or protein can strain the kidneys, particularly in individuals with CKD.

4. **Interactions with Medications:**
    - Herbal supplements can interact with prescription medications, potentially causing harmful side effects.

Overuse of Vitamins

While vitamins are essential for health, excessive intake of certain vitamins can harm the kidneys.

1. **Vitamin C:**
    - High doses can lead to kidney stones due to increased oxalate production.

2. **Vitamin D:**
    - Excessive vitamin D can cause calcium buildup in the kidneys, leading to calcification and damage.

How Stress and Lack of Sleep Can Impact Kidney Health

The connection between mental and physical health is well-established, and kidney health is no exception. Chronic stress and inadequate sleep can contribute to kidney damage through various pathways.

Stress

Stress triggers physiological responses that can negatively affect kidney function over time.

1. **Elevated Blood Pressure:**
   - Stress causes a temporary spike in blood pressure, and chronic stress can lead to sustained hypertension, a major risk factor for CKD.

2. **Hormonal Imbalance:**
   - Stress hormones, such as cortisol and adrenaline, can disrupt kidney function by altering fluid balance and increasing inflammation.

3. **Lifestyle Choices:**
   - Stress often leads to unhealthy behaviors, such as poor diet, smoking, or excessive alcohol consumption, which further harm the kidneys.

4. **Increased Risk of Diabetes:**
   - Chronic stress can contribute to insulin resistance, increasing the risk of diabetes, a leading cause of kidney disease.

Lack of Sleep

Sleep is essential for the body's repair and restoration processes. Chronic sleep deprivation has profound effects on kidney health.

1. **Disrupted Kidney Function:**
    - Sleep deprivation affects the kidneys' ability to regulate blood pressure, fluid balance, and waste removal.

2. **Increased Risk of CKD:**
    - Studies show that individuals who consistently sleep less than six hours per night are at a higher risk of developing CKD.

3. **Hormonal Dysregulation:**
    - Poor sleep disrupts hormones that regulate kidney function, such as aldosterone and antidiuretic hormone (ADH).

4. **Weakened Immune System:**
    - Insufficient sleep impairs the immune system, increasing susceptibility to infections, including kidney infections.

The Role of Sleep Apnea

Sleep apnea, a condition characterized by interrupted breathing during sleep, is particularly harmful to kidney health.

1. **Reduced Oxygen Supply:**
    - Frequent drops in oxygen levels strain the kidneys and increase the risk of damage.

2. **Linked to Hypertension and Diabetes:**
    - Sleep apnea is closely associated with these conditions, compounding the risk of CKD.

Practical Strategies to Protect Kidney Health

Addressing harmful lifestyle habits is essential for preserving kidney function and preventing complications. Here are actionable strategies:

Quit Smoking

- Seek support through counseling, nicotine replacement therapies, or smoking cessation programs.
- Replace smoking with healthier habits, such as exercise or meditation.

Limit Alcohol Consumption

- Follow guidelines for moderate drinking: up to one drink per day for women and two drinks per day for men.

- Opt for alcohol-free alternatives when socializing.

Stay Hydrated

- Drink plenty of water throughout the day to prevent dehydration.

- Monitor urine color as an indicator of hydration levels.

Use Medications Responsibly

- Follow recommended dosages and avoid prolonged use of NSAIDs or PPIs.

- Consult a healthcare provider before starting any new supplements or medications.

Manage Stress

- Practice relaxation techniques, such as deep breathing, yoga, or mindfulness meditation.

- Engage in regular physical activity to reduce stress levels.

Prioritize Sleep

- Aim for 7-9 hours of sleep per night.

- Create a sleep-friendly environment by keeping the bedroom dark, quiet, and cool.

- Address sleep apnea or other sleep disorders with medical intervention.

Lifestyle habits significantly impact kidney health, often in ways that are not immediately apparent. Smoking, excessive alcohol consumption, dehydration, misuse of medications, and chronic stress or sleep deprivation can all contribute to kidney damage and disease progression. Recognizing these risks and making positive changes can protect your kidneys and improve overall health.

By quitting harmful habits, staying hydrated, using medications responsibly, and prioritizing stress management and sleep, you can take proactive steps to safeguard your kidneys for the long term. Kidney health is not just about treatment but also prevention—and adopting healthy lifestyle choices is a powerful way to achieve that goal.

CHAPTER 8

Natural Remedies and Preventative Measures

The health of your kidneys is a cornerstone of overall well-being. While medical advancements have provided effective treatments for kidney-related issues, natural remedies and preventative measures can play a significant role in supporting kidney function and preventing disease. This chapter explores herbs and supplements that may benefit kidney health, tips for maintaining kidney wellness at different life stages, and the role of exercise in promoting kidney function.

Herbs and Supplements That May Support Kidney Function

Certain herbs and dietary supplements have shown promise in promoting kidney health and preventing complications. However, these remedies should always be used under medical supervision to avoid interactions with medications or adverse effects.

1. Dandelion Root

Dandelion root is a natural diuretic, which can help promote urine production and support the kidneys in flushing out toxins.

- **Benefits:**
    - Reduces water retention.
    - Supports detoxification processes.
- **Usage:**
    - Typically consumed as a tea or supplement.

2. Nettle Leaf

Nettle leaf is rich in antioxidants and anti-inflammatory compounds, making it beneficial for kidney health.

- **Benefits:**
    - Reduces inflammation in the urinary tract.
    - May help prevent kidney stones.
- **Usage:**
    - Brewed as a tea or taken as a capsule.

3. Cranberry

Cranberry is well-known for its role in preventing urinary tract infections (UTIs), which can ascend to the kidneys if untreated.

- **Benefits:**
    - Prevents bacteria from adhering to the urinary tract walls.
    - Reduces the risk of recurrent infections.
- **Usage:**
    - Consumed as unsweetened juice or in supplement form.

4. Turmeric

Turmeric contains curcumin, a powerful anti-inflammatory and antioxidant compound that may benefit kidney health.

- **Benefits:**
    - Reduces inflammation in chronic kidney disease (CKD).
    - Protects against oxidative stress.

- **Usage:**
    - Added to food, consumed as a tea, or taken as a supplement.

5. Milk Thistle

Milk thistle is primarily known for its liver-protective properties but may also benefit the kidneys by reducing inflammation and oxidative damage.

- **Benefits:**
    - Supports detoxification.
    - Protects kidney cells from damage.
- **Usage:**
    - Taken as a supplement or brewed into tea.

6. Omega-3 Fatty Acids

Omega-3 fatty acids, commonly found in fish oil, are essential for reducing inflammation and protecting kidney function.

- **Benefits:**
    - Lowers blood pressure, reducing strain on the kidneys.

- Supports cardiovascular health, indirectly benefiting the kidneys.

- **Usage:**

    - Consumed through fatty fish (e.g., salmon, mackerel) or supplements.

7. Vitamin D

Vitamin D is crucial for maintaining healthy bones and regulating calcium-phosphorus balance, functions closely tied to kidney health.

- **Benefits:**

    - Prevents calcium buildup in the kidneys.
    - Supports immune function.

- **Usage:**

    - Obtained through sunlight exposure, fortified foods, or supplements.

8. Ginger

Ginger has anti-inflammatory and antioxidant properties that can benefit kidney health, particularly in individuals with diabetes or CKD.

- **Benefits:**
    - Reduces inflammation.
    - May help regulate blood sugar levels.
- **Usage:**
    - Consumed fresh, as tea, or in supplement form.

Precautions with Supplements

While many herbs and supplements offer potential benefits, some can be harmful if taken in excessive amounts or by individuals with pre-existing conditions. Always consult a healthcare provider before adding supplements to your routine, particularly if you have CKD or are on medication.

Tips for Maintaining Kidney Health at Different Life Stages

Kidney health requirements change throughout life. Adapting your lifestyle to meet these changing needs is essential for preserving kidney function at every stage.

1. Childhood and Adolescence

Promoting healthy habits during childhood and adolescence lays the foundation for lifelong kidney health.

- **Hydration:**
  - Encourage children to drink water regularly to prevent dehydration and UTIs.
- **Diet:**
  - Provide a balanced diet rich in fruits, vegetables, whole grains, and lean proteins.
- **Physical Activity:**
  - Encourage regular exercise to support overall health.
- **Avoid High-Sodium Foods:**
  - Limit processed snacks and fast food.

2. Adulthood

As the body matures, the kidneys may face increased strain from lifestyle factors, work stress, and dietary habits.

- **Manage Blood Pressure and Blood Sugar:**
  - Monitor and control these levels to prevent CKD.

- **Limit Alcohol and Tobacco Use:**
    - Both habits can impair kidney function over time.
- **Routine Checkups:**
    - Regular blood and urine tests can detect early signs of kidney issues.

3. Pregnancy

Pregnancy places additional demands on the kidneys, making it crucial to prioritize kidney health during this time.

- **Stay Hydrated:**
    - Proper hydration supports increased blood volume and kidney workload.
- **Monitor Blood Pressure:**
    - Pregnancy-related hypertension can lead to complications.
- **Balanced Diet:**
    - Focus on nutrient-dense foods that support both maternal and fetal health.

4. Older Adulthood

The risk of kidney disease increases with age. Adopting kidney-friendly habits becomes even more important.

- **Stay Active:**
    - Regular physical activity helps maintain healthy blood flow to the kidneys.
- **Monitor Medications:**
    - Be cautious with NSAIDs and other medications that may harm the kidneys.
- **Reduce Protein Intake:**
    - In individuals with declining kidney function, excessive protein can strain the kidneys.

Exercise and Its Connection to Kidney Wellness

Physical activity benefits not only cardiovascular and mental health but also kidney function. Regular exercise helps maintain optimal blood flow, regulate blood pressure, and support overall health, indirectly protecting the kidneys.

1. Benefits of Exercise for Kidney Health

- **Improved Blood Pressure:**
    - Regular aerobic exercise helps lower high blood pressure, a major risk factor for CKD.

- **Better Blood Sugar Control:**
    - Exercise increases insulin sensitivity, reducing the risk of diabetes-related kidney damage.

- **Weight Management:**
    - Maintaining a healthy weight alleviates pressure on the kidneys.

- **Reduced Inflammation:**
    - Exercise helps lower systemic inflammation, which can damage kidney tissues.

- **Enhanced Circulation:**
    - Improved blood flow supports kidney filtration and overall function.

2. Types of Kidney-Friendly Exercises

1. **Aerobic Exercise:**
   - Activities like walking, cycling, swimming, or dancing improve cardiovascular health and blood pressure control.

2. **Strength Training:**
   - Light resistance exercises build muscle mass and enhance metabolism without overstraining the kidneys.

3. **Yoga and Stretching:**
   - These activities promote relaxation, reduce stress, and improve circulation.

4. **Low-Impact Activities:**
   - For individuals with mobility issues or CKD, low-impact exercises like tai chi or water aerobics provide gentle benefits.

3. Precautions for Exercising with Kidney Issues

- **Hydration:**
  - Drink water before, during, and after exercise to prevent dehydration.

- **Monitor Intensity:**
    - Avoid overexertion, as excessive strain can lead to dehydration or increased blood pressure.

- **Consult a Physician:**
    - Individuals with CKD or other medical conditions should consult their healthcare provider before starting a new exercise regimen.

Natural remedies and preventative measures are invaluable tools for maintaining kidney health and preventing disease progression. Incorporating kidney-supporting herbs and supplements, adapting health strategies to different life stages, and engaging in regular exercise can significantly enhance kidney function and overall well-being.

By taking a proactive approach to kidney health, you can reduce the risk of developing chronic kidney disease and other complications. Whether through mindful dietary choices, tailored exercise routines, or the use of natural remedies, these preventative measures empower you to take control of your health and safeguard your kidneys for the future.

CHAPTER 9
Living with Kidney Disease

Living with kidney disease can be a life-altering experience that demands both physical and emotional resilience. Whether you have been diagnosed with chronic kidney disease (CKD) or another kidney condition, managing the challenges associated with the disease requires a comprehensive approach. This chapter explores how to cope with a diagnosis, the available treatment options, including dialysis and transplantation, and the emotional and psychological aspects of managing chronic kidney issues.

Coping with a Diagnosis of CKD or Other Kidney Conditions

Understanding the Diagnosis

Being diagnosed with a kidney condition, particularly CKD, can feel overwhelming. CKD is a progressive disease that ranges from mild kidney impairment to complete kidney failure. Early stages often go unnoticed, as symptoms can be subtle or non-existent. Receiving a diagnosis, therefore, can come as a shock to many patients.

1. **Gather Information:**
   - Educating yourself about your condition is an empowering first step. Understanding what CKD is, how it progresses, and its potential complications can help you feel more in control.
   - Ask your healthcare provider about your stage of CKD, your glomerular filtration rate (GFR), and any specific markers like proteinuria.

2. **Work with a Healthcare Team:**
   - Your healthcare team may include a nephrologist, dietitian, social worker, and primary care physician. Together, they will create a tailored care plan to address your medical needs and lifestyle goals.

3. **Develop a Support System:**
   - Family and friends can play a crucial role in providing emotional and practical support. Joining a kidney disease support group can also connect you with others facing similar challenges.

Adjusting to Lifestyle Changes

Living with CKD requires making adjustments to protect your kidney health and overall well-being.

1. **Dietary Changes:**
    - Work with a dietitian to create a kidney-friendly diet. This may involve reducing sodium, limiting protein, and managing potassium and phosphorus intake.

2. **Hydration:**
    - Follow your doctor's recommendations on fluid intake. Too much or too little water can strain the kidneys.

3. **Medication Management:**
    - Take prescribed medications as directed and avoid over-the-counter drugs that can harm the kidneys, such as NSAIDs.

4. **Routine Monitoring:**
    - Regular checkups and lab tests are essential to track your kidney function and adjust your treatment plan as needed.

Treatment Options: Dialysis and Transplantation

When kidney disease progresses to end-stage renal disease (ESRD), treatment options like dialysis or a kidney transplant become necessary to sustain life. Understanding these treatments can help you make informed decisions.

Dialysis

Dialysis is a procedure that performs the kidney's essential function of filtering waste, toxins, and excess fluids from the blood.

1. **Types of Dialysis:**

   - **Hemodialysis:**
     - Blood is filtered through a machine and returned to the body.
     - Sessions typically occur three times a week at a dialysis center, each lasting 3-5 hours.

   - **Peritoneal Dialysis:**
     - A dialysis solution is introduced into the abdominal cavity, where it absorbs waste before being drained.

- This method can be done at home and offers greater flexibility.

2. **Pros and Cons:**
    - Hemodialysis provides efficient waste removal but requires frequent visits to a center.
    - Peritoneal dialysis offers independence but demands strict adherence to a sterile technique.

3. **Challenges of Dialysis:**
    - Fatigue, dietary restrictions, and potential complications like infections are common challenges.

Kidney Transplantation

A kidney transplant is the surgical placement of a healthy kidney from a donor into a person with ESRD. It is often considered the best treatment option for eligible patients.

1. **Types of Donors:**

    o **Living Donors:**

    - A kidney is donated by a living relative or friend.

    o **Deceased Donors:**

    - Kidneys from deceased individuals are matched to recipients on a transplant list.

2. **Benefits of Transplantation:**

    o Restores nearly normal kidney function.

    o Eliminates the need for dialysis.

    o Improves quality of life and life expectancy.

3. **Challenges of Transplantation:**

    o Lifelong immunosuppressive medications are required to prevent organ rejection.

    o The risk of infection and side effects from medications must be managed carefully.

    o Wait times for a suitable donor can be lengthy.

4. **Eligibility:**
   - Transplant eligibility depends on overall health, age, and the presence of other medical conditions.

Emotional and Psychological Aspects of Managing Chronic Kidney Issues

Living with a chronic condition like CKD is not just a physical challenge—it also has significant emotional and psychological implications. Addressing these aspects is critical to maintaining overall well-being.

Emotional Impact

1. **Shock and Denial:**
   - A diagnosis of CKD often brings feelings of disbelief and denial. Patients may struggle to accept the reality of their condition.

2. **Anxiety and Depression:**
   - Uncertainty about the future, financial concerns, and lifestyle changes can lead to anxiety and depression. These feelings are particularly common during the early stages of the disease or when starting dialysis.

3. **Grief:**
    - Many patients experience grief over the loss of their previous health and lifestyle. This can include feelings of anger, frustration, and sadness.

Coping Strategies

1. **Seek Professional Help:**
    - A counselor, psychologist, or psychiatrist can provide strategies for managing stress, anxiety, and depression.

2. **Join Support Groups:**
    - Connecting with others who understand the challenges of living with kidney disease can provide comfort and practical advice.

3. **Mindfulness and Relaxation Techniques:**
    - Practices like meditation, deep breathing, and yoga can reduce stress and improve emotional resilience.

4. **Stay Informed:**
   - Understanding your condition and treatment options can reduce feelings of helplessness and empower you to take an active role in your care.

Family and Social Dynamics

1. **Communicate Openly:**
   - Share your feelings and concerns with loved ones to foster understanding and support.

2. **Set Boundaries:**
   - Manage expectations around what you can and cannot do, especially during treatment phases like dialysis.

3. **Maintain Social Connections:**
   - Staying connected with friends and participating in social activities can combat isolation and improve mental health.

Maintaining a Positive Outlook

1. **Focus on What You Can Control:**
    - Adhering to your treatment plan, eating a kidney-friendly diet, and staying active can give you a sense of control over your health.

2. **Celebrate Small Wins:**
    - Acknowledge progress, such as stable lab results or successful dialysis sessions.

3. **Set Realistic Goals:**
    - Break larger objectives into smaller, achievable steps to maintain motivation.

Practical Tips for Living with Kidney Disease

1. **Create a Routine:**
    - Establishing a daily schedule for medications, meals, and treatment sessions can provide structure and reduce stress.

2. **Stay Active:**
    - Regular physical activity, tailored to your abilities, can improve energy levels and overall health.

3. **Track Your Progress:**
    - Keep a journal of your symptoms, lab results, and how you're feeling to identify patterns and improvements.

4. **Plan for Emergencies:**
    - Have a list of medications, healthcare providers, and emergency contacts readily available.

Living with kidney disease presents numerous challenges, but it is possible to lead a fulfilling life with the right approach. By understanding your condition, exploring treatment options, and addressing emotional and psychological needs, you can take proactive steps to manage your health and maintain a high quality of life.

Whether you are navigating the early stages of CKD or undergoing dialysis or transplantation, a supportive healthcare team, a strong personal support network, and a positive mindset can make all the difference. Remember, you are not alone—resources and support are available to help you every step of the way.

CHAPTER 10

Healthier Lifestyle to Prevent Kidney Problems

Your kidneys are among the most vital organs in your body, working tirelessly to filter waste, balance fluids, and regulate blood pressure. Protecting their health requires a combination of proactive lifestyle choices, regular medical care, and inspiration from those who have successfully improved their kidney function. This chapter outlines actionable steps for a healthier lifestyle, emphasizes the importance of medical checkups, and shares inspiring stories of individuals who overcame kidney challenges to live fulfilling lives.

Steps for a Healthier Lifestyle to Prevent Kidney Problems

Preventing kidney problems begins with adopting habits that support overall health. A kidney-friendly lifestyle can reduce the risk of chronic kidney disease (CKD) and other kidney-related complications.

1. Maintain a Balanced Diet

Eating a balanced diet is one of the most effective ways to protect your kidneys. A diet rich in nutrients and low in harmful substances can reduce the strain on your kidneys and improve their function.

- **Limit Sodium Intake:**
    - High sodium levels can increase blood pressure, putting extra stress on the kidneys.
    - Opt for fresh foods over processed ones and use herbs and spices instead of salt for flavor.

- **Control Protein Consumption:**
    - Excessive protein intake can overwork the kidneys. Stick to moderate portions of lean proteins like fish, chicken, and plant-based sources.

- **Monitor Potassium and Phosphorus:**
    - People with kidney concerns should be cautious with high-potassium foods (bananas, potatoes) and phosphorus-rich foods (dairy, processed meats).

- **Incorporate Antioxidant-Rich Foods:**
  - Berries, leafy greens, and citrus fruits can help reduce inflammation and oxidative stress in the kidneys.

2. Stay Hydrated

Water is essential for kidney health, aiding in waste removal and preventing the formation of kidney stones.

- Aim for 8-10 cups of water daily unless your doctor advises otherwise.
- Monitor the color of your urine; clear or light yellow is a good indicator of proper hydration.
- Avoid excessive consumption of sugary or caffeinated beverages.

3. Exercise Regularly

Physical activity supports cardiovascular health, which directly impacts kidney function.

- **Aerobic Exercise:** Activities like walking, cycling, or swimming improve circulation and blood pressure regulation.

- **Strength Training:** Builds muscle mass and promotes metabolic health without overburdening the kidneys.

- **Yoga and Stretching:** Help reduce stress and improve blood flow.

- Aim for at least 150 minutes of moderate-intensity exercise per week.

4. Avoid Smoking and Excessive Alcohol

- **Smoking:**
  - Damages blood vessels and reduces blood flow to the kidneys.
  - Increases the risk of CKD and kidney cancer.

- **Alcohol:**
  - Excessive drinking dehydrates the body and increases the risk of high blood pressure, which strains the kidneys.

5. Manage Chronic Conditions

- **Diabetes:**
  - Keep blood sugar levels under control to prevent diabetic nephropathy, a leading cause of CKD.

- **Hypertension:**
  - Regularly monitor and manage blood pressure to protect the kidneys.

- **Obesity:**
  - Maintaining a healthy weight reduces the risk of kidney disease and related complications.

6. Be Cautious with Medications

- Avoid long-term use of nonsteroidal anti-inflammatory drugs (NSAIDs) like ibuprofen and naproxen, as they can harm the kidneys.

- Always follow your doctor's advice regarding over-the-counter medications and supplements.

7. Reduce Stress

Chronic stress can contribute to high blood pressure and kidney problems. Incorporate stress-relief techniques such as:

- Deep breathing exercises.
- Meditation or mindfulness practices.
- Spending time in nature or engaging in hobbies.

The Importance of Regular Medical Checkups

Why Regular Checkups Matter

Routine medical checkups are critical for detecting kidney problems early and preventing complications. Many kidney conditions, including CKD, progress silently without obvious symptoms until significant damage has occurred.

1. **Early Detection:**
    - Regular tests can identify markers like high creatinine levels, proteinuria, or declining glomerular filtration rate (GFR).

2. **Monitoring Chronic Conditions:**
   - Regular visits allow for better management of diabetes, hypertension, and other conditions that impact kidney health.

3. **Preventive Care:**
   - Doctors can provide personalized advice on diet, exercise, and medications to protect your kidneys.

Key Tests for Kidney Health

1. **Blood Tests:**
   - Measure creatinine levels and estimate GFR to assess kidney function.

2. **Urine Tests:**
   - Detect protein or blood in the urine, which may indicate kidney damage.

3. **Blood Pressure Monitoring:**
   - High blood pressure is both a cause and a consequence of kidney disease.

4. **Imaging Tests:**

- Ultrasound or CT scans may be used to detect structural abnormalities in the kidneys.

When to See a Nephrologist

Consult a kidney specialist if:

- You have persistent protein or blood in your urine.
- Your GFR is consistently below 60 mL/min.
- You have a family history of kidney disease or other risk factors.

Inspiring Stories from People Who Improved Their Kidney Health

1. Rachel's Journey to Reversing Early CKD

Rachel, a 45-year-old teacher, was diagnosed with stage 2 CKD during a routine health checkup. Shocked by the news, she decided to make significant lifestyle changes.

- **Dietary Changes:**
    - Rachel worked with a dietitian to adopt a low-sodium, plant-based diet. She replaced processed snacks with fresh fruits and vegetables and reduced her protein intake.

- **Increased Physical Activity:**
    - She began walking 30 minutes daily and gradually added yoga to her routine.
- **Medical Monitoring:**
    - Regular checkups and lab tests showed gradual improvement in her GFR over two years.

Rachel's commitment to her health allowed her to reverse the progression of CKD and regain her confidence.

2. James's Triumph Over Hypertension-Related Kidney Damage

James, a 60-year-old retired engineer, struggled with uncontrolled hypertension for years. When his doctor detected declining kidney function, James knew he had to act fast.

- **Medication Adherence:**
    - James began taking his prescribed blood pressure medications consistently.

- **Lifestyle Modifications:**
    - He quit smoking, reduced alcohol consumption, and followed a DASH (Dietary Approaches to Stop Hypertension) eating plan.
- **Stress Management:**
    - Meditation and gardening became his go-to stress relievers.

James's efforts paid off, and his kidney function stabilized, allowing him to avoid dialysis and enjoy his retirement.

3. Maria's Recovery After a Kidney Transplant

Maria, a 38-year-old nurse, developed end-stage renal disease (ESRD) due to lupus. After spending three years on dialysis, she received a kidney transplant from a living donor—her sister.

- **Post-Transplant Care:**
    - Maria followed her immunosuppressive medication regimen diligently to prevent rejection.

- **Adopting Healthy Habits:**
    - She maintained a balanced diet, exercised lightly, and stayed hydrated.
- **Finding Purpose:**
    - Maria now volunteers with a kidney disease awareness organization, sharing her story to inspire others.

Maria's resilience and gratitude have fueled her mission to live a full and meaningful life.

Protecting your kidneys is a lifelong journey that requires consistent effort and informed decision-making. By embracing a healthier lifestyle, prioritizing regular medical checkups, and drawing inspiration from others who have improved their kidney health, you can take control of your well-being and reduce the risk of kidney disease.

The roadmap to healthy kidneys begins with small, actionable steps: eating a balanced diet, staying active, managing stress, and seeking medical care when needed. Remember, the choices you make today can have a profound impact on your kidney health and quality of life in the years to come. Let the stories of triumph and resilience shared in this chapter motivate you to take the first step on your journey to optimal kidney health

CONCLUSION
Kidney Health Is a journey

Your kidneys are the unsung heroes of your body, working tirelessly every day to maintain balance and support life. Through their filtration of blood, regulation of electrolytes, and removal of waste, they perform vital tasks that are often taken for granted. However, as this book has illustrated, kidney health is not guaranteed and must be actively preserved. From understanding the anatomy and functions of the kidneys to recognizing the warning signs of trouble, the journey to kidney wellness begins with awareness and informed choices.

The chapters in this guide have explored the complexities of kidney health, detailing common problems, preventative measures, and treatment options. As we conclude, it's essential to revisit the core lessons and emphasize the steps that will empower you to take control of your kidney health for a better quality of life.

Recognizing the Silent Threats

One of the most important takeaways from this book is that kidney diseases are often silent. Chronic kidney disease

(CKD), for example, can develop over years without noticeable symptoms. This underscores the importance of routine medical checkups and early detection. Simple tests like blood creatinine levels, glomerular filtration rate (GFR), and urine protein analysis can reveal much about your kidney function. By staying vigilant and addressing issues early, you can significantly reduce the risk of severe complications.

Beyond CKD, conditions like kidney stones, infections, and acute kidney injury (AKI) highlight how diverse kidney problems can be. Each of these conditions has unique symptoms, risk factors, and treatment options, but they all share a common thread: the potential to escalate if ignored. This book has provided a detailed understanding of these conditions to help you identify them and seek timely care.

The Role of Lifestyle in Kidney Health

The health of your kidneys is deeply intertwined with your daily habits. The choices you make in your diet, physical activity, and stress management play a pivotal role in either supporting or straining your kidneys.

Diet and Hydration

As discussed, a kidney-friendly diet is low in sodium, balanced in protein, and mindful of potassium and phosphorus levels. Incorporating antioxidant-rich foods like berries, leafy greens, and whole grains can help reduce inflammation and oxidative stress. Hydration is equally critical; drinking enough water helps prevent kidney stones and ensures efficient filtration. However, moderation is key—overhydration can be just as harmful as dehydration.

Avoiding Harmful Substances

Smoking, excessive alcohol consumption, and the overuse of certain medications, such as NSAIDs, can significantly harm the kidneys. These habits damage blood vessels, strain kidney function, and increase the risk of chronic conditions like hypertension and diabetes, both of which are leading causes of kidney disease. Quitting smoking and moderating alcohol intake are vital steps toward preserving kidney health.

Physical Activity and Weight Management

Regular exercise supports cardiovascular health, which directly benefits the kidneys. Physical activity helps regulate blood pressure, improves insulin sensitivity, and promotes weight management—all factors that reduce the risk of kidney disease. Engaging in activities like walking, swimming, or yoga can be both enjoyable and effective in maintaining overall wellness.

Managing Chronic Conditions

For those living with chronic conditions such as diabetes or hypertension, managing these diseases is critical to preventing kidney complications. High blood sugar levels and elevated blood pressure are two of the most common causes of kidney damage. This book has provided strategies to manage these conditions, from medication adherence to lifestyle modifications. By keeping these chronic issues under control, you can significantly reduce your risk of kidney problems.

Understanding Treatment Options

Despite the best preventative measures, some individuals may face advanced kidney disease requiring dialysis or transplantation. This book has outlined these treatment options to demystify what can be an intimidating process.

- **Dialysis:** While dialysis is life-sustaining, it comes with physical and emotional challenges. Understanding the types of dialysis, such as hemodialysis and peritoneal dialysis, empowers patients to choose the method that best fits their lifestyle.

- **Kidney Transplantation:** A transplant offers the potential for a renewed life but requires careful consideration of eligibility, donor matching, and post-transplant care. For many, the benefits outweigh the challenges, offering improved quality of life and freedom from dialysis.

Learning about these treatments helps individuals make informed decisions when faced with advanced kidney disease.

Emotional and Psychological Resilience

Living with kidney disease affects more than just the body; it also impacts the mind and emotions. Coping with a diagnosis, undergoing treatments, and managing lifestyle changes can lead to feelings of stress, anxiety, or even depression. Recognizing these emotional aspects is essential for holistic care.

This book has highlighted the importance of:

- Building a support system of family, friends, and healthcare providers.

- Seeking professional counseling or joining support groups for shared experiences and encouragement.
- Practicing mindfulness, meditation, or other relaxation techniques to reduce stress.

By addressing the psychological challenges of kidney disease, individuals can enhance their overall well-being and resilience.

Inspiring Stories of Kidney Recovery

Throughout this guide, real-life stories have showcased the power of determination and proactive care in overcoming kidney challenges. These stories serve as reminders that kidney disease, while serious, is not insurmountable. With the right mindset, medical support, and lifestyle changes, it is possible to live a fulfilling life even with a kidney condition.

The Importance of Community and Advocacy

Improving kidney health extends beyond individual efforts. Advocating for kidney awareness, supporting research, and fostering community connections can create a broader impact. Whether through donating to kidney-related organizations, participating in awareness campaigns, or sharing your story, you can contribute to a collective effort to reduce the burden of kidney disease globally.

Final Thoughts

A healthy life begins with informed choices and proactive care. Your kidneys are resilient, but they require attention and care to function at their best. By applying the knowledge from this book, you have the tools to protect your kidneys, prevent potential problems, and navigate any challenges that arise.

Remember, kidney health is a journey, not a destination. Whether you're adopting preventative measures, managing a chronic condition, or exploring treatment options, each step you take brings you closer to a healthier, more balanced life. Let this guide be a constant resource and inspiration as you prioritize your kidney health and overall well-being.

Your journey to kidney health starts today. Take the first step, and know that your efforts will make a lasting difference—not just for your kidneys, but for your entire body and mind.

www.ingramcontent.com/pod-product-compliance
Lightning Source LLC
Chambersburg PA
CBHW050306230526
45471CB00005B/2049